"A heart-warming and inspiring true tale that captures the human spirit of love and caring. Christian was so fortunate to have found those qualities in Mrs. Sirdashney. One dedicated teacher truly can make a difference in the lives of so many."

DEBORAH LUPIA
Former Principal, School Five

"*Cranes for Christian* is such a heart-warming and touching story. Erica was able to capture Christian's true spirit, his personality, and how much he was loved. *Cranes for Christian* leaves you with a smile, just like Christian always did."

STEPHANIE L. FOOKS-PARKER, MSW LSW
& DR. STEPHAN GRUPP MD, Ph.D.

"Regardless of your walk of life, regardless of whether or not you or someone you love is dealing with a terminal illness, this book is a must-read. The encouragement and hope it will bring will reach deep into your situation and touch you. As a pastor to Christian for most of his life, I can say that through his illness, and even in his death, he was an example of what true Christianity is. He never complained, always smiled, was more concerned about others than himself, and I admire him to this day for it."

PASTOR AMIR M. KHAN

Cranes for
CHRISTIAN

———◆———

For Lisa,
Much love,
Erica Svidashney

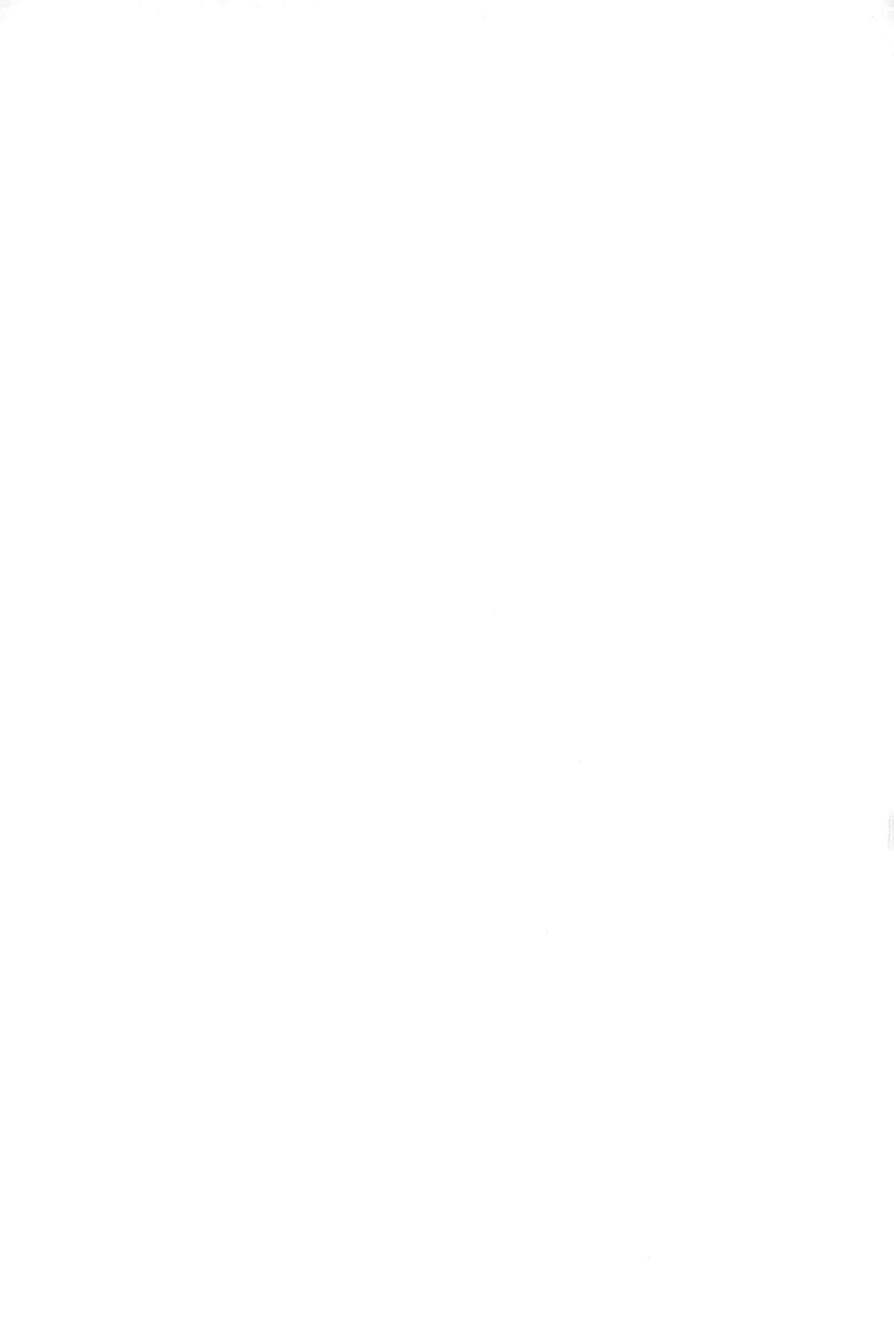

Cranes for CHRISTIAN

ERICA SIRDASHNEY

Tate Publishing & Enterprises

The opinions expressed by the author are not necessarily those of Tate Publishing, LLC.

Published by Tate Publishing & Enterprises, LLC
127 E. Trade Center Terrace | Mustang, Oklahoma 73064 USA
1.888.361.9473 | www.tatepublishing.com

Tate Publishing is committed to excellence in the publishing industry. The company reflects the philosophy established by the founders, based on Psalm 68:11,
"The Lord gave the word and great was the company of those who published it."

Published in the United States of America

ISBN: 978-1-60462-788-6
1. Family & Relationships: Death and Grief

08.03.10

This book is dedicated to Christian,
the boy who always had a smile on his face.

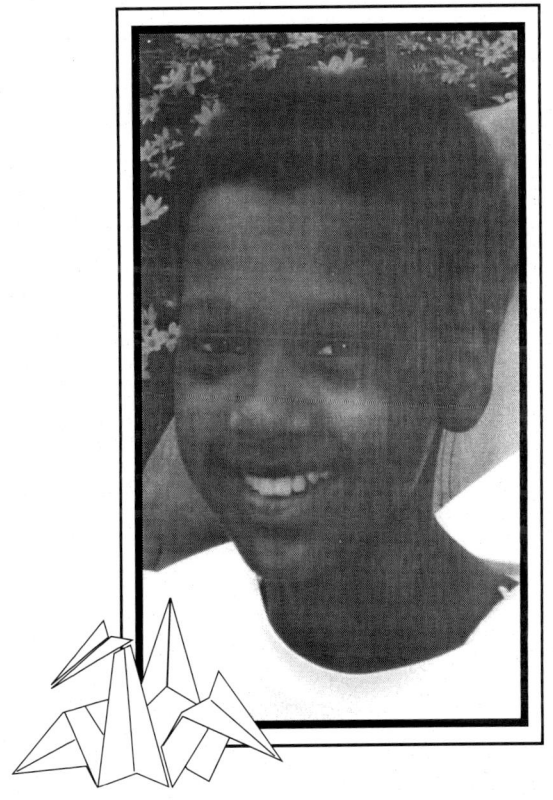

ACKNOWLEDGMENTS

Thank you, Eileen. Thank you, School Five. None of this would have been possible without your love, support, and involvement. And to my grandmother in heaven, who always believed in my abilities and insisted I was a writer: thanks, Nanny!

TABLE OF CONTENTS

FOREWORD

God's timing is always the right timing. Our family stood witness to this. After many years of battling cancer, Christian was ready to accept the fact that he was going to die. School Five extended themselves to us in such a gentle and loving manner. It was overwhelming for us to receive. When the entire school rallied around Christian, it gave him the strength to fight harder and make it through his final round of treatments. The cranes really helped to lift his spirit. Oftentimes, I would find him lying in bed, watching the cranes, crying. Christian knew how special it was for his classmates, friends, and school community to do something like that for him.

Christian also knew that he had some very special teachers at School Five, in particular, his third grade teacher Erica Sirdashney. Erica is a blessing from God, who spreads the love of God to everyone who is fortunate enough to cross her path. She knew how to get the best out of Christian. He knew she was someone he could believe in and trust. Erica's experiences with cancer enabled her to relate to Christian on a more personal level. Their relationship was by far a work of God. This is evident throughout the entire book. *Cranes for Christian* is the perfecting of God in, with, and through them both.

EILEEN CLARK
Christian's Mom–Mom

INTRODUCTION

"Everything happens for a reason." If I had a penny for every time someone told me that, I'd be rich by now. However, I'd be even richer if I had a penny for every time I said that to someone else! This is a statement I believe in with my whole heart. It's not always easy to do though. You see, even though everything happens for a reason, we don't always know what that reason is. For some of us, that reason comes with time. For others, we may leave this earth never knowing. But for a very few, that reason becomes apparent almost immediately. I consider myself one of these fortunate individuals. I know everything happens for a reason. I know because of Christian.

ARE YOU MRS. SIRDASHNEY?

A re you Mrs. Sirdashney?"

It was the first day back for teachers and we had in-services all day long at the high school. I was on my way back to the auditorium when I was stopped in the hallway.

"Yes, I'm Mrs. Sirdashney."

I extended my hand to greet the woman. Her face was familiar; her voice was familiar. I recognized her as someone I had seen many times before, but I wasn't quite sure who she was.

"I'm Eileen Clark. My grandson Christian is going to be in your third-grade class this year."

Eileen spoke for a few minutes before we parted ways, but what she said, to this day, I cannot tell you. My mind was racing. I couldn't believe that this child was being placed in my room. Christian Clark was very sick. He was diagnosed with cancer years prior and the doctors didn't think he would make it much longer. Truth be told, doctors didn't even know how he was still living. Certainly his blood levels, chest x-rays, and diagnostic testing would support otherwise.

Just a few days prior, while setting up my classroom for the school year, our building principal, Mrs. Lupia, came in to see me. Mrs. Lupia was the one who told me about Christian and his placement in my class. She and the child study team felt it was best. Ordinarily I would have been flattered in their confidence, but something held me back. All I kept thinking was, *How could they do this to me? This little boy has terminal cancer. Chances are he is going to die very soon, and they sent him to me? What were they thinking?*

School Five was where I got *my* phone call. Never in all of my years at School Five had I ever been taken from class for a phone call. It simply wasn't done. And to receive the call in the computer lab while class was in session? What could be so important?

It was my doctor. I went to see the dermatologist because of some rough patches of skin on my arms. I was hoping she had some suggestions for me. Instead, she became focused on a spot I had on my leg. It was a spot I had my entire life. I never thought much of it. I'm covered with spots just like it! The only thing that made it different was its size. Over the past year it had changed, but so did the rest of my body. Pregnancy does that. I just figured it got bigger because my leg got bigger. The doctor did not seem as convinced. She took it for biopsy.

Last I heard the biopsy came back inconclusive. Being that I was young and otherwise healthy, the doctor did not seem overly concerned. Even still, she asked if she could resubmit my sample to another pathologist for further review.

She was pretty sure it was fine, but wanted to be completely sure before sending me on my merry way. A week or so had gone by without word. I assumed no news was good news. Well, you know what they say about people who assume.

"Melanoma."

My results were in. The doctor needed me to schedule my surgery immediately. She also wanted me to contact my primary care physician. Over and over again, the doctor kept telling me she was sorry. She was sorry it took so long, sorry it turned out to be melanoma. However, she then stressed how glad she was that she had indeed sent my sample out again, commenting on what a disaster it could have been if the cancer had gone undetected, untreated.

I made my way up to the main office to contact my husband. Mrs. Lupia met me halfway. I told her about my phone call. The next thing I knew, I was in her office using the principal's private line to call home. When I got off the phone I turned to head back to the lab to pick up my students. That's when Mrs. Lupia stopped me.

"Why don't you have Mike come pick you up?"

"That's okay. I'm fine. I'm going to stay."

I saw no reason why I couldn't go on teaching for the remainder of the day. That's when she said it.

"Erica, I think you need to go home and grieve this."

Grieve this? What did she mean grieve this? I was being sent home? This was ridiculous! Contrary to what others advised, I got in my car and drove myself home. My house, being only a ten-minute drive, if that, didn't give me too much time to think. The first five minutes were devoted to thoughts of how silly I felt for leaving school. It was as if I was playing hooky, leaving school for faking an illness! Although, after revisiting Mrs. Lupia's last comment in the midst of my thoughts, I immediately shifted for the remaining five minutes.

"You need to go home and grieve this."

What did she mean by *grieve* this? What a word to use! Had she done so inappropriately, or was there really something to grieve? Should I be grieving something? Will people grieve me? My goodness, it's not like I could die from this ... could I? That was the one thought that remained present in my mind until I reached home, where my husband was waiting in the driveway. School had called to tell him I was on my way, and now he greeted me with a hug.

Within minutes of getting settled I was on the phone with my primary care physician. I told her the results of my biopsy, and she asked me to come in. Her office was directly across the courtyard from the dermatologist. I could go see my primary care physician, and then head over to the dermatologist's office to schedule my surgery. At this point it didn't seem like such a big deal to me, and I still couldn't understand why people were so concerned. Then I had the talk.

"It's not like I could die from this, right?"

And my doctor sat down…

After a brief silence, she went on to talk about skin cancer.

"Yes, it's true. If you're going to get cancer, skin cancer is usually the best to have…unless it's melanoma."

That's when the doctor went on to explain that melanoma was known as the silent but deadly cancer. Unlike other skin cancers, melanoma has the ability to enter the blood stream. If the melanoma had done so, if it had already metastasized, I would have anywhere from months to seven years to live. That's why it was so important for me to have the surgery. They needed to cut the cancer out before it could get any deeper. It really was a matter of life or death.

Months or seven years? My daughter was only a year old! If I was really sick, if this cancer had entered my bloodstream and best case scenario, I had seven years remaining, Faith would be eight years old when I died. Eight years old! The children I teach are eight years old. How terribly ironic! I teach third grade, and by the time my child is in third grade I could be gone. I couldn't schedule my surgery soon enough.

Within days, the surgery was done—a centimeter around and a centimeter under the original biopsy site. I was awake for the procedure, but didn't mind. My leg looked horrible, but I could care less. I didn't want what was there. They could have it! I just wanted my life back. If only it was that easy…

The second biopsy came back with clear margins, indicating that they got it all. The melanoma, Clarks Level II malignant melanoma, appeared to be rather thin. Chances were good that it had not reached the blood stream; however there was no way of telling without additional diagnostic testing. They checked my lymph nodes, my liver, and my lungs. Those were the places melanoma was known to attack first. The first round of testing went well. My second round of testing came three months later in September; the same time Christian was placed in my third grade class!

This was all hitting a little too close to home for me. I had cancer. Now a child in my class had cancer? Clarks Level II malignant melanoma. Christian Clark? Was this a sign of some sort? Was I going to die? Would this child die while under my care? Oh, to be a student in that class. Could you imagine losing a classmate and a teacher all in one year? That was my biggest fear.

What were they thinking? How on earth was I going to be able to pull this off? Only time would tell.

FLUFFY HAIR

I don't know what I expected Christian to look like when I first met him. One of the child study team members told me Christian had some skin discoloration on his face as a result of previous cancer treatments, but other than that, I wouldn't have even known who he was. Clearly this was not a child who was sick. Clearly this child would not be dying any time soon! He looked healthy as a horse and boy, oh boy, was he happy. It didn't matter what time of day it was or what we were doing in class, Christian always had a smile on his face. And nothing made him smile more than his fluffy hair.

Third grade was one of the first years Christian had hair again. During his earlier years at School Five, he lost his hair due to the cancer treatments. Over the summer it had grown back, and as I found out later in the year, Christian had no desire to cut it. The fluffier, the better! I cannot tell you how many times I would be in the middle of a lesson when out of the corner of my eye I would spot Christian patting his hair. The smile on his face! It was as if he just needed to check and see that it was still there.

Each day Christian came to school, Mrs. O'Donnell,

one of our special education teachers stopped by to see if Christian needed help with his work. Mrs. O'Donnell had worked with Christian each year. If Christian was absent or he wasn't feeling up to the work, Mrs. O'Donnell would often take him to her room. Although he was quite fond of Mrs. O'Donnell and he looked forward to her checking in each day, Christian never left the room. He was staying put.

As time went by I started to forget that Christian had cancer. Coincidentally, I seemed to forget about my cancer as well. It was as if his happiness was contagious. You couldn't help but feel good when Christian was around you. He was just such a happy, positive kid! There were times I wondered if the doctors could be wrong. I had just about convinced myself of that fact when Mrs. Lupia came for another visit.

Christian was a patient at the Children's Hospital of Philadelphia, also known as CHOP. Arrangements had been made for one of the counselors from CHOP to come in and talk to the third graders about Christian's cancer. Time was set aside and classes were doubled up for a brief program of sorts. I didn't think much of it until the program began and the counselor started talking about Christian's cancer and what he goes through on a daily basis. It was important for the children to understand that even though they had to be careful around Christian because of his port, the place where his medication is administered during treatments, they did not have to worry about catching Christian's cancer. It was not contagious.

The last couple of minutes of the program were devoted to student questions. When the counselor asked the students if they had any questions about what she had shared, or questions about Christian's cancer, I found myself exchanging knowing glances with the other classroom teacher and Mrs. Lupia. Would anyone dare to ask it? Would anyone ask if Christian was going to die?

I hoped, for his sake, they did not. After all, he was in the room with everyone else. Although he did not look upset by any stretch of the imagination, he was not wearing his trademark smile at the time. He was clearly uncomfortable with the attention he was receiving. In fact, when the counselor asked if he wanted to tell the kids anything about his cancer and his experiences at CHOP, Christian's response was a very quick, but quiet, "No."

Would we make it through the presentation without the question being asked? One by one, the hands went up, the questions were asked, answered, and the hands went down. We were just about done when one hand remained. Up, down, up, down, then up again.

"Did you have a question in the back?"

"Umm … yeah … Can cancer kill you?"

There you had it. The question we all feared. For as much as I feared the question, at least the thought of it lingered in my mind. I was prepared to hear it. What I was not prepared for was the answer. It hit me like a line drive to the kneecaps.

"Well, kids usually don't die from cancer. Most of the time it's adults who die from cancer."

I froze in my seat. I felt my principal's eyes upon me, but I could not turn to meet her glance out of fear that if I did, I would well up and cry. That's when her hand touched my shoulder.

"Why don't you go take a walk and get yourself something to drink."

I suddenly realized how brave Christian was when he very quickly, but quietly said no to his counselor's question. Here I was, unable to look my principal in the eye, unable to speak. All I could do was shake my head no. I was not going to leave. Christian sat through the entire presentation like a trooper. There was no way I was going to walk out on him. I was staying.

When the presentation ended, the students were given a small activity to complete and the adults were called out into the hallway. We discussed how well the students did and we thanked the counselor for her time. As I turned to go back into my classroom the counselor reached out to stop me.

"I think we all need to prepare ourselves …"

My heart sank into my chest, and my eyes welled up uncontrollably.

"Christian's cancer is getting worse. At this point in time, there's nothing else that can be done for him. The doctors don't expect him to make it through the holidays."

Easter

After our private session with the counselor from CHOP, I had prepared myself for the worst. What I had feared more than anything was going to come to pass. I was going to lose this little boy while he was under my care. I thought of the children in my class, especially the kids who were so close to him. What would they do when they lost him? I thought about his grandmother, the one who is closest to him, the one who loves him and cares for him day in and day out. How horrible for her to suffer such a loss! Would she ever be able to enjoy the holidays again?

And yes, I thought about me. I thought about my cancer and my testing. Clearly this had to be a sign. So often Christian would go for blood work, and I would go for blood work. Christian would have his lungs checked, and I would have my lungs checked. There must have been a reason for us to be brought together under these circumstances.

As difficult as it was, I continued to smile each and every day. Christian wore his trademark smile as well. The smile looked great in our Halloween pictures. He smiled even bigger when Mrs. Sirdashney gobbled like a turkey the entire week before Thanksgiving. Christian went on to smile through

Hanukkah, Christmas, and Kwanzaa! Before we knew it, it was the New Year, and do you know what? Christian smiled real big when I said, "Happy New Year, buddy!"

He wouldn't make it through the holidays? Well, maybe they were talking about Easter, because the holidays had just passed and Christian was still with us. He wasn't going anywhere. In fact, I really started to believe in what Christian's grandmother Eileen had once told me.

"They can tell me he's going to die all they want. I know different. Christian is a fighter and he's not going anywhere."

Time and time again, hadn't he done just that? He wouldn't make it to first grade ... Definitely not through second grade ... As for third grade with me, he wasn't even supposed to make it through the holidays! Well Happy Easter, enjoy your Spring Break. Christian is still with us. Still smiling, still patting his fluffy hair, still refusing the extra help because he didn't need it.

I no longer feared Christian. I no longer feared cancer. I no longer feared losing him. I embraced it all. Clearly there was a reason for Christian to enter my life, and I was open to it. Let him fight. I'll fight with him! Christian was not going anywhere. Christian was going to finish third grade with Mrs. Sirdashney.

A SECRET

The school year was just about over when Christian suffered a bit of a setback. His tumors were growing, and they were spreading rapidly. They were causing pain and often prevented him from eating. Together with the doctors, the decision was made to go for surgery. Would the surgery cure his cancer? No, but we were hoping it would at least provide some relief.

As the date grew nearer, Christian really started to struggle. I noticed changes in his behavior, and Eileen had reported that he was not eating or sleeping very well.

"If he's having difficulty getting through the day, send him to the nurse's office to rest, or give me a call and I'll come pick him up."

To say that Christian was tired would be an understatement. His head rested on his hands all morning. His eyelids were heavy, dark rings circled below them, and I hadn't seen that trademark smile in several days. I half expected him to nod off at any moment. Every once in a while I would quietly ask if he was okay.

"Do you need to go to the nurse?"

He immediately perked up, smiled, and said, "No."

"Are you sure you don't want me to call Mom-Mom to come and get you?"

He shook his head vehemently. "I don't need to go home. I want to stay here."

Well, maybe he would finish out his day at School Five, but I did not feel comfortable sending him out for recess. Surely that would do him in. Knowing Christian the way that I did, he'd never admit to being uncomfortable, so I decided to find a way to avoid the situation entirely.

"Would you like to be my special helper today?

With a nod and flash of that trademark smile I had been missing for so many days, I knew we were in business. Christian agreed to stay in for recess to help me out with my mailboxes. Thank goodness he did not suspect a thing. In addition to not admitting his level of discomfort, Christian was not one to readily accept help or pity either.

As the students lined up to go to recess, I handed Christian a stack of notices. One by one he placed them in the mailboxes. Before the last student could file out the door, Christian was done.

"What's next?"

I had nothing for him. I paused awkwardly, scanning the room for the next task. Christian followed my gaze around the room, but then he began to focus in on me. I could see the pieces of the puzzle being put together in his mind. He knew what I was doing, and he wasn't happy about it in the slightest.

"Christian, why don't you come and sit down with me at the reading table for a minute. I want to talk to you about something."

The reading table is a table located in front of my desk. Students often meet in groups for guided reading practice. We also conduct writing conferences at that table. Come to think of it, students are called to the table numerous times throughout the day. To be invited is an honor indeed. Sometimes we run out of chairs. However, as a class we always agree that if one can stand and wait quietly, participating where appropriate, you can stay and wait for the next chair to open up. The students love that table. I have to admit, I do as well. It's a good place to be.

So here we were, sitting at the table, and it was just the two of us. Christian didn't have to wait for a seat to become available. He didn't even have to share me with a group. Rather than taking my usual seat at the head of the table, we sat across from one another. It appeared that this was a little too much for Christian to take. Clearly the suspense was getting the best of him.

"Can I tell you a secret?"

That did it! Not only did Christian light up like a light bulb, but he was now leaning so far across the table, his bottom barely touched the seat.

He smiled and nodded yes.

"Christian, you have shared so many of your secrets with me over the past couple of months. I thought it was about time I shared one of mine with you."

I went on to tell Christian about my cancer. I told him how I got the phone call at School Five just that past spring. I told him how scared I was, how I was afraid that I wouldn't be around to teach the kids or raise my daughter. I told him about my surgery and how they had to cut out a portion of my leg. I told him many times when he was going for bloods, I was going for bloods. He was getting his lungs checked and I was getting my lungs checked. It seemed we had a lot in common, and now that he was preparing for his surgery, we had even more in common than before.

I made sure to tell Christian that our cancers were very different. So far all I needed was surgery. The doctors felt the surgery had helped my cancer; it may have taken it all away for good! I then went on to say that it was my hope that his surgery would help his cancer, just like my surgery helped me.

At first he just stared at me. I asked if he had any questions for me. Clearly he did, but was in need of permission before doing so. Once given the clearance, he asked question upon question upon question. I answered them the best I could. I then asked him about his surgery. Did he want to tell his classmates about it? Did he want me to tell them about it? He asked if I would tell them once he was in the hospital. I agreed to do so, and before I knew it, it was time to bring the class back in. I thanked Christian for his help. He just smiled.

Later that week I received a call from Christian's grandmother, Eileen. She said she didn't know what I had done or what I had said, but whatever it was, it worked like a charm. Christian was eating, Christian was sleeping, and he was more than ready for his surgery.

The day finally arrived and Christian went in for his surgery. Per his request, I told the students about it after his departure. I explained that he would need much time to heal and we probably wouldn't see him for several weeks. The class was given some time to make cards for Christian, and we agreed we would continue to make cards and write letters each week he was away from School Five. Believe it or not, we only sent out one set! Not because we were too busy, and not because we forgot, but because we were not given the opportunity to send more. I received a call from Eileen.

"Erica, are you ready for this?"

I braced myself, not knowing what to expect.

"He's coming back, Erica. He wants to come back to school. He says he feels fine; he doesn't want to stay home anymore and he's coming back to school tomorrow."

And that's exactly what he did, trademark smile and all! Regardless of any report the doctors may have given, I knew Christian's surgery was a success. Eileen and the doctors supported Christian's decision to come back to school. They were amazed at his recovery and his ability to heal so quickly. However, as time went by, we were all beginning to realize that nothing should surprise us as far as Christian was concerned.

Here's one thing that did surprise me though: Several months, if not a year or so later, Eileen and I had a conversation about the days leading up to Christian's surgery. We talked about him not eating, we talked about him not sleeping, and I talked a bit about the conversation we had the day he stayed in to help during recess. Do you know Eileen never knew? She really had no idea what we discussed! She didn't know about my cancer. She didn't know about any of it! I assumed he would have told her, but he didn't. I still remember saying to Eileen repeatedly, "He really didn't tell you?"

She went on to explain that he told her about helping out, and he told her about us having a talk of sorts, but he would not go into details. Eileen tried to get it out of him several times, but his reply was always the same, "It's a secret, Mom-Mom."

CARE PACKAGES

I have an aunt and her name is Lorraine, but to anyone who knows her, family or not, she's Aunt Raine. Aunt Raine is my mother's youngest sister. She is not married and she does not have children. When I was a child I often wondered why God did not give her a family of her own. Aunt Raine would make such an amazing mother! Then again, God only knows what I'd be and where I'd be without her. Aunt Raine is one of the very special people in life. I think one of the things that makes her so amazing is the fact that there are countless other people in the world who would say the very same thing.

When I was a child, I decided I wanted to grow up to be just like Aunt Raine. I wanted to keep a clean house. I wanted to take lots of pictures and make albums. I wanted to do special things for people. Most of all, I wanted to make people feel as special as Aunt Raine always makes me feel. There are many ways to do that.

Aunt Raine is a good listener. She takes interest in your life and who you are. She knows what you like, what you don't like, and the reasons why. She knows your friends, the ones you love, and the ones who have hurt you. Because Aunt

Raine knows you so very well, she knows just what to do and say to make you feel special.

Whenever I was in a concert or a show at school, Aunt Raine was always there to cheer me on. She usually had a little gift to mark the occasion too. For me, it was anything with a star on it. My self-esteem was never very strong, and this was Aunt Raine's way of reminding me that I was indeed a star.

When I spent weekends with her or stayed overnight, we always made a trip to the grocery store first. She took me down the junk food aisle and I got to pick out my favorite snack, even if it was the brand name kind. I still remember eating my snacks out of that little orange Tupperware container. This snack in the bright orange container represented so much! It was a representation of the love and the care that was given so freely. The love and care I so desperately needed.

As I got older the events in my life changed, as did my little gifts from Aunt Raine. A trip to the shore found a new, crisp, white night gown to sleep in on a warm summer night. When I was away at college, it was a card every now and then telling me to consider myself hugged. Inside was a ten-dollar bill with a note to go out and get a pizza or something with my friends. And how could I ever forget the day that Mike and I brought our daughter Faith home from the hospital? Wasn't Aunt Raine there to celebrate that a new *star* was born?

No matter how old I am or what the life situation, Aunt Raine always knows what to do and what to say to make me feel special. She has gone on to do so for my children, reminding me each and every day how it's done. So much of who I am today is because of Aunt Raine's influence in my life. So much of what I do, what I say, and how I care for others is the direct result of the example she has set.

That's how care packages came to be. You see Christian *did* finish third grade with me, but his summer was a long one, a hot one, and a difficult one. Often the heat was too much for him and he could not go outside to play because he had difficulty breathing. How heartbreaking it was for him. Christian loved the outdoors. Whether it was camping, fishing, or riding bikes with Mom-Mom, outside and active is what Christian wanted to be. What made matters even more difficult was the fact that he lived with a cousin who was the same age, and Jamal could play outside and wanted to be outside all the time. This made Christian feel terrible.

My first care package arrived during this time. Since Christian couldn't go outside, I had to find something that would occupy his time and keep him interested indoors. I went to the craft store and picked up some art supplies. There were markers and crayons, doodle pads, puzzles, and stickers. I threw in some Silly Putty as a bonus. Silly Putty was the coveted item in Mrs. Sirdashney's third grade class.

After the craft store I went to the bookstore. I picked up some of Christian's favorite chapter books, as well as some riddles and rhymes to pass the time. My last stop was the grocery store for one or two of Christian's favorite snacks. Once I had it all together, I went to the post office, packed it all up in a large box, and mailed it off to Christian, who lived five minutes away from my house. Did you really think I'd do it any other way? Think about it, how did you feel when you got mail as a kid?

A phone call from Eileen and Christian told me it was indeed a hit. Not only was Christian enjoying his care package, but Jamal was too! The boys were having such fun together, neither of them thought about missing the outdoors. Jamal wanted to be inside with Christian, and Christian didn't have to feel guilty about keeping Jamal away from other activities. Do you know, out of everything in that first care package, Christian's favorite was the boogy-eye stickers? They probably cost me all of ninety-nine cents, if that, but as I mentioned above when I spoke about Aunt Raine, it's never about the money, is it? It's about the love and the care you give. It's about knowing someone well enough to be able to brighten their day. It's all about the way you make them feel. And do you know the best part? If you do it right, the feeling returns to you ten fold. I know because I learned from the best.

CRANES FOR CHRISTIAN

I continued to put together care packages for Christian throughout the summer and into the new school year. He was in Mrs. Renner's fourth grade class and still full of surprises. The doctors said he would not be able to walk much longer, as it was becoming more and more difficult for him to breathe. They suggested the use of oxygen and a wheelchair or motorized scooter to get from place to place while at school. Christian would not hear of it. He walked in line with the rest of his class, never falling behind, but occasionally pausing to meet my glance as I passed in the hallway. A tap here, a pat on the shoulder there, just a little something to let him know that he was still my buddy. However nothing over the top that would embarrass him in front of his friends.

Fourth graders were the oldest in the building, you know. It wasn't exactly cool to be best friends with a teacher. Although I may not have been the recipient of that trademark smile, a little sideways smirk was the reminder that we still shared a special bond, a special secret.

During the holiday season I was away from School Five. As usual, I started with a cold, which led into bronchitis, and landed me home in bed with pneumonia. I cannot tell you how many times this has happened to me. I've grown rather used to it, as have the people who know and love me best. Very rarely am I at School Five around the holidays.

Christian was at school though. His class, like many others, was celebrating the holiday season as well as the upcoming winter break. It was a neat time of year, especially if you were a kid. This was the time of year when one could say, "See you next year!" and get such a kick out of it. The statement was sure to fool a few who heard it. To anyone in school, you often think of the year as starting in September and ending in June. So when you say, "See you next year," there's always those who think of the next school year rather than a few days after the break when we all return in January.

Well, it was during Christian's party and during these statements that Christian traveled down a path he had never cared to venture before. When his classmates were going back and forth telling each other, "See you next year," Christian told a small group of his classmates they would not see him next year. In fact his exact words were, "You will not see me next year because I am going to die."

I was not there to hear this statement, but I know it word for word because of the phone call I received after the holidays. It was Mrs. Renner, Christian's fourth grade teacher. He was back at CHOP and when Mrs. Renner asked if there was anything she could do for him, his response was, "Would you tell Mrs. Sirdashney where I am?" So that's what she did. She told me where he was and she told me about the conversation that had taken place during his class party. I was devastated.

In all the time I had known Christian, I never heard him speak that way. Eileen said it best when she said that Christian was a fighter. Medically speaking, there was nothing to support his being able to sustain life. But that's because medicine was not keeping Christian alive. Christian was keeping Christian alive. His tremendous spirit was what kept him and everyone around him going.

With him saying he was going to die, I knew he had given up, and that scared me. Where was that hope? Where was that fighting spirit? More importantly, what, if anything, could I do to help get it back? That's when I prepared for my first visit to CHOP. That's when I prepared the care package I am most proud of to this day.

At the time I had no idea what I was going to do, no idea what I was going to say. I just went about my business of picking up a little of this and a little of that. However, while at the bookstore I was struck with a sudden thought. There was a book. A book about a young girl who was sick with cancer. She had given up her battle just as Christian had given up his. Then there was something about a paper crane. The crane symbolized hope, a wish to be granted to one who was dying. I knew this all not because I read the book, but because my cooperating teacher, mentor, and good friend from School Five had once told me about it. Joyce Braddock read that story to each of her third grade classes year after year. If only I could remember the name of the book!

Sadako! Sadako and the Thousand Paper Cranes! That was the story and that was the book I so desperately needed. I found myself feverishly searching for it. Up and down the aisles I went until I found it and added it to my stack of books already selected. Yes, this was the book I needed. This was the book that was going to change it all. My care package was complete. Or so I thought…

When I arrived home that night, I sat down to read the book. A short read, it did not take me long to finish it cover to cover. As I sat and read, the story became more and more meaningful. With each turning page I was reminded of Christian. This was his story. He, like Sadako, had cancer. He, like Sadako, was a fighter. However, he, like Sadako, had given up hope. The crane represents hope. Sadako's best friend made her first crane. I could make Christian's. Others could join me. If he had given up hope, we would hope for him. We would make his thousand cranes. We would restore his hope and help grant his dying wish.

It all started with one crane. One crane I did not know how to make!

The instructions for making a paper crane are in the

back of the book. The instructions list thirty-three steps. I gathered a piece of white computer paper, fashioned it into a square, took a deep breath and went about following the instructions, one step at a time. As I sat on the floor at the glass coffee table in my living room, I was suddenly brought back to my childhood. My best friend Mia is of Japanese decent. How many times had we sat and done origami together as children? Yet, how many times was I able to successfully make a crane? Never! In all my years, I never made a crane. It was the most difficult origami figure to master!

Although fold after fold, my crane started to take shape. No sound escaped my lips, but I could feel tears streaming down my face. I was overcome with emotion. I was making a crane. I was doing it. I was so proud. What's more, I knew what this symbolized; I knew what this meant for Christian. Step thirty-one … Step thirty-two … Step thirty-three! I was done and it was beautiful! I had successfully made a crane and I couldn't stop there. I went on to make crane after crane after crane until my husband told me it was time to go to bed.

The next morning I woke up bright and early. In the back cover of *Sadako*, I wrote a message to Eileen. I wrote of my plans for Christian. I understood he had given up hope, and that was okay. We were going to hope for him. We were going to make his thousand cranes and I had the first one to present to her that day. She could share it with Christian. She could tell him what it was all about.

During the ride into the city that day I sat very quietly, which was unusual for me. Usually I'm a bit of a chatterbox. I couldn't speak because I was deep in thought. My husband, Mike, asked me if I was okay repeatedly. Each time I nodded silently, retreating back into my private thoughts. Shortly before our arrival however, I perked up.

"Cranes for Christian!"

"What?"

"Cranes for Christian, Mike. That's what we're going to call it! *Cranes for Christian*!"

THE SCHOOL FIVE FAMILY

School Five is indeed a family. There's no doubt about it. You will never find a more caring group of professionals. In addition to taking care of our students, we reach out to their families, the community, and we take care of each other as well. Whenever anyone is in need, whenever there's cause for celebration, School Five is there. That's why I knew I could reach out to them when it came to Cranes for Christian.

Eileen was completely touched by the book and the paper crane. A former student had given her a box of cranes in the past, but she did not know the story of *Sadako*, nor was she familiar with the legend behind the paper crane. To say that Eileen approved of my plan for Christian was putting it lightly. She too was at a loss. It was not like Christian to behave this way. He was giving up. He was giving in to it all.

Christian was just so, so sad, and he was incredibly tired. Worst of all was the pain. His tumors were growing so large; they were causing unbearable discomfort. The new plan was to prepare Christian for a final round of radiation. In a matter of days he would be placed under isolation. The period of isolation would lead into radiation. During this time, Eileen talked to Christian about *Sadako and the Thousand Paper Cranes*.

While Eileen was sharing with Christian, I was already contacting my family at Five. First was the building principal. I told her about my visit to CHOP. We discussed Christian's condition and my plan regarding the cranes. She backed me one hundred percent. When we returned back to school after the winter recess, our first faculty meeting was devoted to Cranes for Christian.

I knew Mrs. Lupia put some time aside for me to speak, so I typed something up to bring with me. I couldn't get through it. As much as I wanted to, as excited as I was to introduce this project, I just couldn't get the words out. Mrs. Lupia took over for me, reading what I had planned to present to the faculty and staff. By the time she was done, there was not a dry eye in the house. People who knew Christian, people who knew of Christian, people who knew nothing of Christian—all were on board.

I went out to every craft store I could find to purchase origami paper. Mrs. Lupia gave me a personal check to help fund the project, as did many others. Photocopies of the thirty-three step instructions were distributed, and I provided lessons before and after school, during my prep, and at lunch. Those who felt confident enough to do so went on to instruct others. There were even a few who went on to instruct their classes.

Before we knew it, the entire school was involved. *Sadako and the Thousand Paper Cranes* traveled around the building, and teachers shared the book with their classes to reinforce the meaning of what we were doing. Of course, there was a post-it in the copy we all shared, advising teachers where to stop the reading and begin the folding. Those who were familiar with the story understood exactly why. The children embraced it. Even the parents and community members became involved in the effort. This is the poem that hung in our main office window for all to see.

Cranes for Christian

One thousand cranes for Christian
Each folded with a prayer
Filled with hope and love and joy
To show him that we care!

Each day that Christian remained in isolation, preparing for his last round of radiation, we collected cranes. My classroom was the drop-off zone. What a sight to see—bins, bags, and baskets of cranes coming through the door one after the other after the other. We made a large pile on the floor in the front of the room. Together as a class, we counted the cranes. Once we were done, we buzzed the office with the total. The total was announced over the loudspeaker and the whole school cheered. Then a call was placed to CHOP. Each day the total was posted on a sign in Christian's window to let him know what was accomplished on behalf of him.

Do you know that in just three short days we reached our goal of one thousand cranes? In fact, we surpassed it! Children continued to fold cranes in class, during recess, and at home each night. Teachers and staff members continued to fold cranes with the students, on their own, and with family members at home. They kept coming and coming, each new set more beautiful, more unique. We had large cranes, small cranes, and itty-bitty baby cranes. We had cranes made from origami paper, construction paper, notebook paper, and yes, even cranes made from the occasional missing homework assignment! It was amazing.

What was even more amazing was the fact that it seemed to be working. Christian's spirits were lifting. How could they not? He had a whole school, a whole community, a whole family behind him. Everyone was thinking about him. Everyone was hoping and praying for him. His cranes were done. One thousand cranes for Christian! All he needed to do now was make a wish. Anything he wanted. It was his for the asking. His for the taking.

CHRISTIAN'S WISH

What Christian wanted more than anything was to finish the year at School Five. Our district being an extremely transient one, it was rare for students to attend kindergarten through fourth grade. Yet Christian had been with us each and every year so far. Fourth grade was the last grade level in our building. Christian desperately wanted to come back. School Five was his family. In fact, I believe School Five was in many ways the family God truly intended for Christian.

If Christian was going to make it back to School Five, he needed to be well enough to go home first. In order to get well, Christian needed to eat. This was not an easy task for Christian. Just the thought of food often made Christian sick to his stomach. He couldn't look at it, he couldn't tolerate the smell of it, and he definitely was in no position to ingest it. Any time he made the attempt, it came right back up anyway. No one understood this feeling better than I did.

When I was just a few weeks pregnant with my daughter, Faith, I suffered a dog bite. It was so early in the pregnancy, we didn't even know for sure if I was pregnant at the time. Still, we proceeded cautiously. I was given an antibiotic to ward off any possible infection. The antibiotic was safe to take during pregnancy. It was not however safe for me.

Shortly after the drug was administered I became violently ill. My symptoms were dismissed as morning sickness. I was sent to the emergency room countless times to receive IV fluids. At one point I could not even tolerate water. I was placed on home IV therapy. It didn't work. I was losing more and more weight with each passing day.

At my worst, I was finally admitted to the hospital. It wasn't until my fourth month of pregnancy that a young ER physician figured out what was truly wrong with me. By that time, I was so completely filled with toxins, I was told, "Take this medication or you and your baby are going to die."

The antibiotics tackled the toxins in my system, but that still left me with the nausea and vomiting. Four months of nonstop nausea and vomiting! Compazine didn't work. Reglan didn't work. Phenergan didn't work either. Those are the main drugs used to combat nausea and vomiting. Each time the drugs were administered the doctors told me I would experience immediate relief. Well, that never happened. Instead I suffered an allergic reaction known as dystonic reaction. Basically it's like you want to crawl out of your very own skin. The best part? Every time you suffer from dystonic reaction, the episode is more severe than the last. So here I was four months pregnant and my six foot two husband had to put me in a bear hug to keep me from going crazy once again!

A new team of doctors took over my care and I was given a drug called Zophran. It was wonderful. It was my new best friend! However, it was also terribly expensive and difficult to obtain. The insurance company kept denying my claim. The pharmacy could not fill my prescription. I didn't care how expensive it was. I'd take out a second mortgage if I needed to! It was the only drug that offered relief after four months of suffering. I needed it! My baby needed it!

The problem, as they explained it, was Zophran is a drug usually reserved for cancer patients. I was not a cancer patient. How many times were they going to remind me of this fact? Enough times for me to remember when it counted the most.

"Have they given Christian Zophran yet?"

Imagine my surprise when Eileen told me no. Eileen then talked to the doctors and nurses about Zophran. They agreed to give it a try. Slowly but surely, the Zophran started to do its job. Now Christian had to do his. A young child, and one who had suffered so, he was now almost petrified to eat. Discussions at mealtime often erupted into arguments and awkward silences. The nurses tried. The doctors tried. Eileen even gave it her best effort! No one could get Christian to eat. No one that is, except for me.

So for a long time, that became my role in Christian's life.

It was my job to get Christian to eat. My job to help build his strength enough to get him home and back at School Five. But first and foremost, I needed to help rebuild his confidence. He needed to trust me. He needed to trust what I was saying.

"I know it's hard, Christian, but you have to give it a try. The first bite is the hardest. Once you get a little bit of food in your stomach, you'll feel so much better."

He just stared at me. He wanted so much to do what I requested of him. "Christian, I know exactly what you're feeling right now. I know it feels like you're going to be sick, but the Zophran is doing its job. Once you have some food in your belly you won't feel sick anymore, I promise."

I picked up a small dinner roll and handed it to Christian. For a few minutes, he just looked at it. With a short glance back up at me, he brought the roll to his lips and took a bite.

Bite after bite, Christian was eating once again. It wasn't a full recovery of appetite, but it was enough to hold off the threat of a feeding tube. So visit after visit, day after day, that was my job. It was my job to get Christian to eat. No sooner would I walk through that door, than Eileen would say, "Mrs. Sirdashney's here! Time to eat, Christian!"

And he did. Together we surveyed his tray of food, and together we decided which would be best for him to eat that day. With time, he started to pick a little on his own.

He even started eating for others. No lengthy discussions, no arguments! Christian knew what he needed to do. If he wanted out of that hospital, if he wanted to go back home, if he wanted to finish fourth grade at School Five—he had to eat.

I have to admit; it was during this time that I didn't know if Christian would *ever* make it out of the hospital. With him not eating for so long, the doctors started preparing us for the worst. It was suggested to Eileen that she consider hospice. They were unsure how much time Christian had left. So as far as returning to School Five was concerned? Well, that would truly put our cranes to the test!

That's when my husband and I decided to bring the cranes in to show Christian. We entered the hospital, each of us carrying two large, clear storage bins filled to the brim with paper cranes. Needless to say, we received quite the reception that day. Some people asked what we were carrying. Others just stared. Christian's floor—well, that was another story. I'll never forget the response we received. The nurses put their hands over their hearts. With tears in their eyes, they explained that they had *never* seen anything like it! What a tremendous compliment.

Eileen stopped us at Christian's door and told us not to bring all of the cranes in. Even though Christian had completed his radiation treatments, there were still levels of radiation present in the room. Anything brought in would be contaminated and have to be later discarded.

"I want those cranes, Erica. I cannot bear to part with any of them. Please, don't bring them all in."

Per Eileen's request, I brought only a few cranes into Christian's room to share with him. I thought it was important for him to see exactly what had been done. He loved them. I placed a few around the room for decoration. I also placed a few in his doorway. In the center of it all was a copy of the poem that resided in the window of School Five. Now all of CHOP would know about Cranes for Christian as well.

After our visit, Mike and I gathered up the cranes to take them back to School Five. Rather than surrounding Christian with his cranes at the hospital, it was decided that we would set them up at home. However, not all of the cranes, just the first 500. Christian wanted the remaining 500 at School Five. This had become his incentive. He would make it home to see his first 500 cranes. Then he would make it back to School Five to see the remaining.

His wish. His command. He was determined and I no longer questioned it. If Christian said he was coming home, he was coming home. If Christian said he was coming back to school, he was coming back to school! See it was not only Christian who had come to trust what I said, I had come to

trust what he said as well. So I went about making the necessary preparations for each of his arrivals.

STRINGING PARTIES

Upon my word, Christian's family at Five got busy preparing his cranes. It wasn't enough to have all thousand of them folded; I wanted the cranes to fly! Su Lakatosh, our wonderfully talented art teacher at Five, worked with me on a model for others to follow. I knew I wanted to string the cranes up somehow, but I didn't want the string to be in sight. Su suggested a nylon monofilament, similar to fishing wire.

I took one of my famous trips to the craft store and purchased monofilament spools by the dozen. I also purchased several packages of needles. Once I turned the materials over to Su, the true magic took place. It was exactly what I had envisioned. A long strand of cranes, suspended in midair without the slightest sign of what enabled them to do so. They were absolutely breathtaking!

The Stringing Parties took place after school hours. All who were interested in doing so met in the media center to string cranes for Christian. There was a large table for people to sit around while stringing cranes. A few tables were set up with refreshments as a little thank you to those who volunteered their time. The remaining tables were set up with the piles and piles of cranes.

Everyone who entered the media center did so with mouths wide open. And that was only the first 500! The magnitude of what we had accomplished really started to set in. We made it our goal to string all 500 cranes that day. We stayed all afternoon, through the evening, and even into the wee hours of the night, but we did it. There was not one lone crane when we left the building.

From the school, I drove over to Eileen's place. Mike and I went about the business of hanging the cranes. We started hanging them in Christian's room. Eileen was overcome with emotion. Her love of the cranes was apparent from day one when I presented the first to her at the hospital, but to see them in flight? She had to leave the room several times as we were hanging them. Upon one of her returns, I stopped hanging cranes and embraced her. With tear-filled eyes, she thanked us once again for doing all that we had done.

"This is awesome, Erica. He's going to love it!"

After the room was filled with cranes, we went on to decorate the remainder of Christian's home. I placed a small treasure chest of cranes next to Christian's bed as a finishing touch. These were the tiniest of cranes, the most difficult to make, the most precious. I thought he might get a kick out of them and enjoy playing with them from time to time.

Before leaving, I took some pictures of the cranes to share

with the School Five Family. The pictures were posted with the poem in the front office window for all to see. For as beautiful as they appeared to be, the pictures didn't do them justice. But that's okay. All would soon see.

A second Stringing Party took place to prepare the remaining 500 cranes. Believe it or not, the power went out while we were working. Not a light in the entire building, but that didn't stop us! We ventured out of the media center, huddling together under exit signs for the smallest bit of light. What a terrific time we had. A colleague and dear friend of mine stated at a much later date that she never saw a community of people come together so willingly and effortlessly as we did when it came to Cranes for Christian. But then again, how could we not?

After school hours the following day, I asked to borrow Mr. Ron's ladder. I started at the front entrance and made my way down to Christian's classroom. It was as if the cranes were showing the way! A single path that led to a classroom filled with cranes. It was complete. One thousand cranes were in flight. One thousand cranes were waiting for Christian's return.

DINNER DATES

"M y crane made Christian better!"

This is a statement that could be heard in the kindergarten wing, the first and second grade hallway, the third grade hallway, and the fourth grade hallway of School Five. Students all over School Five were talking about their cranes and how they made Christian better. It was difficult to determine who was more excited though, the students of School Five, the teachers and staff, or Christian himself.

You see, not only did Christian make it home from the hospital, but he did indeed make it back to School Five. What's more, he finished his school year, making it the culmination of his academic career—an academic career spent entirely at School Five, just as he wished.

Toward the end of the school year Christian and I decided it was time for us to have a dinner date. All that time in the hospital, we often talked about our favorite foods, the ones we couldn't eat when we were so ill, the ones we couldn't wait to eat when we were feeling better! The number one food choice for both of us was tacos. So that was that! We would have a taco dinner date.

In all the years I taught at School Five, I never invited a student into my home. This was new for me. It's not that I never wanted to, in fact, each and every year there was at least one child in my class, usually an unkempt, neglected, or troubled child that I just wanted to take home to spoil with love and attention. Although these days in education, you're lucky if you get away with a pat on the shoulder, let alone a hug. Taking a child into your home? It just wasn't done!

Nevertheless, plans were made. Christian, Mom-Mom, and Christian's cousin Jamal would be joining us for dinner. I made a special trip to the grocery store to purchase all of the necessary ingredients. Chopped meat, lettuce, cheese, tomatoes, taco shells, tortilla wraps, taco seasoning, and taco sauce. But that wasn't all. On my way up to the register I grabbed a bag of Scoops.

Scoops are tortilla chips, but they're shaped like little bowls. They're good for dipping. They hold a lot of dip. They hold a lot of salsa. They're just the right size for you to pop in your mouth. Yes, Scoops would be perfect for our dinner date.

Christian was eating again, but as I mentioned previously, his appetite was not fully restored. Food was still intimidating at times, especially if it came in large quantities. So I decided in addition to making my traditional tacos, I would prepare a tray of mini-tacos as well. I would create my mini-tacos using the Scoops!

"You're nuts, you know that, don't you?"

Eileen stood in the doorway of my kitchen, watching as I sorted through the bag of Scoops for chips that were not broken. As I selected the chips, I placed them on a large cookie sheet. I then went about filling each Scoop with chopped meat.

Very carefully, I loaded my teaspoon with a small portion of meat. With another teaspoon, I coaxed the meat off the spoon, into the tortilla chip. It was working out beautifully. It would take me a good amount of time, but that was not my concern.

"You have the patience of a saint!"

Eileen was all smiles as I continued to work. When each Scoop was filled with meat, I reached for the cheese.

"Oh, come on!"

Now Eileen had broken into fits of laughter. We both laughed as I one by one placed the individual pieces of shredded cheese over the meat.

"They're tacos, Eileen! They need cheese!"

Christian and Jamal were outside playing in the yard with Mike and Faith. A hot day, we had filled up the pool earlier just in case the boys wanted to swim or cool off. Jamal dove right in. Christian was content to just sit and watch all that was going on around him.

When dinner was ready I called everybody in to eat. The

table was filled with a wide array of taco options. Jamal and Mike went straight for the soft shells. Both of them stuffed the wraps so full they could barely close the tortilla, let alone get it into their mouths. We laughed at them as the contents of their tacos dropped back onto their plates. Clearly, this was not the meal for good manners!

Eileen and I went for the hard shells. Together with the group we talked about the different ways people like to load up their taco shells. Different styles, different orders, different ingredients, different proportions, watching an individual build a taco could be quite telling indeed!

Finally it came time for Christian to make his selection, and as I had suspected, he went straight for the Scoops. Eileen eyed me and smiled. The dinner conversation continued. Mike and Jamal made a mess. Eileen and I crunched away. Faith ate peanut butter and jelly, tacos not being a taste she had yet acquired. Christian returned to the platter time and time again, going back for more of his mini tacos. Eileen and I secretly counted as he ate. It was so hard to contain our laughter, our joy!

After a few minutes, Christian asked to be excused. He retreated to the living room where he curled up on the end of the couch to watch a television program.

"Six! He ate six of them, can you believe it?"

Apparently Eileen and I both wound up with the same total.

As the school year ended and the summer began, we had many more dinner dates as a family. Sometimes we brought food over to Christian. Most times, they came to us. One night Christian wanted to stay overnight. We had a guest-room with a queen-sized bed and Christian knew that was his room whenever he needed or wanted it.

Unfortunately, Eileen could not stay. She had early morning plans the following day and told Christian they would stay over another time. To our surprise, Christian's response was that he would stay without her! A night without Mom-Mom? No way! Mom-Mom was lucky if she could go five feet away from Christian, let alone travel into another room. Yet here he was insisting that he wanted to stay, and he would stay without Mom-Mom. Even still, we agreed to do so another night.

"You are loved," was Eileen's response as they left that night.

"The feeling's mutual." I responded as I hugged her good-bye.

LATE NIGHT PHONE CALLS

There are certain people in this world you would not dare to call late at night, early in the morning, or during mealtime. To do so would be considered uncouth, and would most definitely result in social strains. However, there are others to whom these rules need not apply. It doesn't matter what time of day or what the subject matter, the lines of communication are always open.

I had many a talk with Christian and Eileen. At times we discussed trivial things such as lizards, dogs, and fish tanks. I also distinctly remember a late night plea for ice pops. Any time of day, any time of night, there was never a need to worry. Never the need to apologize. In fact, as our relationship grew, the calls increased in frequency, and the subject matter intensified.

One night I picked up the phone to find Eileen in a considerable amount of distress. For whatever reason, Christian had decided that she was not in good health. He worried about her constantly! Here was this young boy with terminal cancer, and he was worried about the health of his Mom-Mom!

What's more, Christian worried about what would happen if his Mom-Mom was no longer around to take care of him. Eileen told him she was fine. She stressed the fact that she was not going anywhere and he had no need for concern. But Christian worried. He worried about where he'd live. He worried about who he'd live with. There was no consoling him. Eileen tried with all of her might.

"Erica, I'm really sorry to do this to you, but Christian wants to know if he could live with you and your family if anything ever happened to me. I know it's a lot to ask, but is this something you'd be willing to consider?"

How ironic that she felt the need to apologize! Didn't she realize what an honor it was to be thought of in that way? I was touched. I was completely touched. I told Eileen Christian had a home with us whenever and if ever he needed one. As far as we were concerned, he was already a part of our family. He need not be concerned or lose sleep over this issue any longer.

Phone calls continued day in and day out. I looked forward to the conversations with Eileen, as well as the ones with Christian. I liked the fact that I seemed to have the answers to their questions each time. It felt good to help find a solution to the problem, to help ease someone's mind.

Then there was a late night phone call like no other. A late night phone call I was not prepared for. This was the late night phone call I will never, in all of my life, forget.

"Erica, Christian is having a really difficult time. I don't know what to do. He wants to know why. Why does he have to die? He wants to talk to you. Could you talk to him, please?"

The next thing I knew, I could hear Christian's strained breathing on the line.

"Hi, buddy. How are you?

No response.

"Are you having a tough night?"

"Yeah…"

"Are you feeling sad?"

"Yeah…"

"I'm so sorry, Christian. I'm so sorry you're going through this. I wish I could tell you why. I wish I could take it all away, but I can't."

"But why do I have to die? Was I bad?"

My heart broke into a million pieces. I said a quick little prayer, asking God to help me find the words. Help me to ease this young mind. Help me heal his little heart and bring some peace in his dying days.

"No, Christian, you were not bad. And you are not being punished. You are a good and loving boy. I think that's what makes this so difficult. And do you know what, Christian? It doesn't seem fair, does it? All around us we see people who are mean and nasty. We see people who do the wrong thing time and time again. People who hurt others… People who hurt themselves … How come they get to go on living their lives and nothing happens to them?"

"Yeah…"

"Well, Christian, the important part to remember is things are not always as they seem. Just because things look good from the outside, doesn't mean they always are. There may be things we don't know. There may be things that take place later on down the line in the lives of those people."

No response.

"Christian, you are a good boy. You are kind and loving. Everyone loves you very much. God loves you very much. I wish I could tell you why but I cannot."

I then talked to Christian about my daughter's name. I told him Mr. Sirdashney and I named her Faith for a very specific reason. We named her Faith because sometimes life can be very difficult and we don't always know why. But for as difficult as it is, we just have to trust that there is a good reason for everything. God has a plan, and He knows what's best for all of us. It doesn't always seem fair, but we have to trust in His plan.

Christian eventually handed the phone back to Eileen. The minute I heard her voice, rather than his I was hysterical. I never cried the way I cried after that late night phone call. I will be forever changed because of that conversation and the questions that were asked of me.

OCEAN GROVE

"W hy? Why did Christian have to go through this? Why did he have to die?"

I was now the one asking the questions. I asked them of my husband. Then I picked up the phone and asked my aunt as well.

"Aunt Raine, I'm sorry to call so late ... "

"No, no, that's okay. What's the matter? Is everything all right?"

I told Aunt Raine about my conversation with Christian. I asked her many of the questions Christian asked me. She did not have the answers either, but then again, I knew that before I picked up the phone to call. Even so, I had to ask. I had to talk to her. You see, Aunt Raine is one of my late night phone calls. She is one I can call any time of the day, with any subject, no matter how trivial or insignificant. She is one I've always gone to when I was hurt. Sometimes you just need the ones you love to know you're hurting. Maybe that's what Christian needed from me that night. Maybe it was his way of saying, "Yes, I am a fighter. Yes, I have done miraculous things. But boy, oh boy, am I hurting!"

Christian was hurting. Eileen was hurting. I was hurting.

Something needed to be done. No mere care package would make this situation better. To do so would be like putting a tiny Band-Aid on a broken leg. It just didn't work; it didn't even make sense! As difficult as it was, I tried to take my thoughts in another direction.

I thought about Christian. I thought about all of our experiences together, all of our other conversations. The conversations in which we shared our feelings with one another: the things we liked, the things we didn't like, the reasons why.

"If you know someone well enough, you have the ability to brighten their day."

Wasn't that true of Aunt Raine? Hadn't I vowed to make that my goal as well? Clearly I could not make this all go away for Christian, but maybe I could *take* him away from it all. Maybe there was something I could do to brighten his day, even if just for one day.

"Aunt Raine, can I take Christian to Ocean Grove?"

We ended our conversation making plans for Christian's trip.

I shared my thoughts with Eileen the following morning. Christian loved to fish. We could take him to Ocean Grove to do some fishing off the pier. Aunt Raine's house was not far from the fishing pier at all. It would work out beautifully!

Eileen was thrilled. I shared our plans with Christian. He was so very excited.

Now that the plans had been made to take Christian to Ocean Grove for a day of fishing, I had to go about making the necessary arrangements. The arrangements such as the actual fishing, I knew nothing about!

I contacted a member of the fishing club. I told him about Christian. I told him about what I had hoped to do. His response was one I most feared. Clearly set in his ways, he did not seem overly receptive to what I was saying. The fishing club had a few hours' time set aside for children who wanted to come out with an adult later in the month. If I wanted to, I could bring Christian then.

I explained to the man that I did not think we could wait that long. Christian was not doing very well. He was now wheelchair bound and in excruciating pain. This trip could not be put off. I asked if there was any other way, if there was any other place I could take him. He had nothing more to offer. As a last ditch effort, we exchanged information. I thanked him for his time, then hung up the phone.

From that point, I called anyone and everyone! I called the town hall. I called the lifeguard post. I called the visitors' center. Could we fish on the beach somewhere? Which beach? What time of day? For how long? No luck. There was nothing I could do to make this happen. I said a quick little prayer.

Within minutes, my phone rang.

"Erica? It's Bill from the fishing club. Yeah … We'll see you on Sunday."

Thank you, Lord!

Everything was set. We would travel to Ocean Grove on Saturday, stay overnight at my aunt's house, and go fishing the following morning. I could barely contain my excitement. Better still, Eileen and Christian were excited as well! We talked about our plans, what to pack, and we planned our menu. This was going to be terrific!

The ride to the shore was a little over an hour. Mike and I drove in our car, bringing along our daughter, Faith. Eileen followed behind us in her car with Christian, bringing along Christian's cousin, Jamal. I hoped the ride was not too much for them. I looked for some sign from Eileen indicating how the trip was fairing. Christian was curled up with a pillow in the front seat. This was his standard in recent days. The pain, being as significant as it was, it was not uncommon to find him in fetal position.

When we arrived at the shore, we got the children settled and I prepared for dinner. Spaghetti and meatball surprise! This was one of the other menu choices we discussed during one of our visits at CHOP. Christian liked spaghetti and meatballs, but had he ever had meatballs with a surprise?

"What kind of a surprise is it, Mrs. Sirdashney?"

For as well as we had come to know each other, for all that we had been through together, to Christian I was still Mrs. Sirdashney. Turns out, I would always be Mrs. Sirdashney.

When all were called to the dining room for dinner, both boys anxiously eyed the spread. Bread, salad, spaghetti and meatballs.

"There's nothing different about these meatballs," Jamal commented.

"Oh?" was my response. "Try one."

As each boy cut into the first meatball with their forks, their faces immediately lit up!

"Cheese!"

There was a small cube of mozzarella baked into each and every meatball.

"Surprise!"

So now they knew. We all laughed as we continued to eat our dinners. Christian ate his spaghetti. He ate his meatball surprise. And he did so wearing that trademark smile the entire time. After all, in addition to the evening's comedy, he was going fishing tomorrow!

Honorary Members

I woke bright and early on Sunday morning. There was so much I wanted to do. So much I needed to prepare in order to make this day a memorable one. Everyone was still sleeping. Mike and Faith were asleep in Aunt Raine's room. Eileen and Christian were asleep in the middle bedroom. Jamal slept soundly in one of the back bedrooms.

Before going into town, a walk of two blocks, if that, I set the table for breakfast. Just in case anyone got up while I was gone, I wanted them to wake to all of their favorites. The only thing missing from the menu was a few extras I would pick up from the bakery that morning.

It was a beautiful day. As much as I had come to fear the sun after my melanoma diagnosis, the way it shined down upon me that morning felt simply divine! I breathed in the salty air. The wind kissed my cheeks as I walked. I was at peace. This was wonderful. The day was going to be absolutely wonderful. I could feel it in my being.

After picking up some doughnuts and fresh rolls at the bakery, I stopped off at the florist. There is a section of the floral shop devoted entirely to tourists. I picked out my favorite Ocean Grove T- shirt and hat for Christian. I wanted to give him a little something to remember the day by.

When I arrived back at the house, all were still sleeping. Shortly after, my husband woke. Neither of us could believe that Eileen and Christian were still sleeping. Not only was it amazing to find them sleeping late, it was amazing that they had slept at all. Most nights they had gone without due to the pain and discomfort Christian now experienced on a daily basis. I was excited for his day of fishing to begin, but the thought of waking Christian from such a peaceful sleep was something I struggled with.

I quietly entered the bedroom and sat at the edge of the bed. The edge of the bed where I was once greeted by a crisp, white nightgown. Was it any wonder that Eileen and Christian found such peace within these walls? Eileen slowly opened her eyes and smiled up at me. She then glanced at the clock. Her mouth hung open in amazement.

"Wow," was Eileen's only verbal response.

We then turned our attention to Christian. I unrolled the T-shirt I purchased for him that morning. I laid it over him on top of the blankets. I then took the hat and gently placed it on his head. His eyes did not open and he did not say a word, but the makings of that trademark smile were beginning to emerge.

It only took us a couple of minutes to get up and going. Although I was told one adult, Eileen and I both planned to accompany Christian to the fishing pier. We were a bit concerned about his condition that morning. He was in a great deal of discomfort. Clearly the pain patch was not bringing any relief. Even still, Christian wanted to go.

We walked to the end of the street and crossed over to the boardwalk. Christian, wheelchair bound, had his Ocean Grove T-shirt on and his fishing pole in hand. He was ready. We were greeted at the gate by an older man who reminded me very much of my grandfather. Slightly hunchbacked, he shuffled his feet as he walked, the brim of his cap, pulled down over the majority of his face. As soon as the gentleman spoke, I recognized his voice from the phone.

"Good morning, Bill, I'm Erica. We spoke on the phone. Thank you so much for having us!"

"Good morning. Good morning. Come on in. Let's see if we can get you started here."

To my relief, his response was a friendly one. I introduced him to Christian and Eileen. He took us through the clubhouse, out onto the fishing pier. It was like entering a whole new world. In all my years, I had never been out on the end of the fishing pier before. The view was breathtaking.

I noticed a few other gentlemen on the pier with us that morning. Members of the fishing club, they all took time to greet us upon our arrival.

"Hello, Christian. How are you feeling this morning?"

"Good."

He lied.

"That sure is a nice fishing pole you got there! Where are some of the places you like to fish with that pole of yours?"

Christian told Bill how he liked to fish in the lake, the pond, and some streams.

"Oh, and I bet that pole is terrific when it comes to fishing in those lakes, ponds, and streams. But, today we're going to give you one of our poles. This is the pole you'll use for your ocean fishing!"

Bill handed the pole to Christian. It was at least double the size of what Christian was holding. I'm sure, to Christian, it was a magnificent sight!

"Before we can let you use one of our poles, we have to make you an honorary member of the Ocean Grove Fishing Club!"

They placed an Ocean Grove Fishing Club hat on his head, and placed the Ocean Grove Fishing Club T-shirt on his lap.

"Now any time you want to come back and do some fishing, you just need to wear that shirt and hat, and we'll know to let you in!"

As an elementary school teacher, I couldn't have done it better myself. I was in awe of their thoughtfulness and consideration.

With his club member's hat on and new fishing pole in hand, we wheeled Christian out to a spot on the pier. A member helped Christian cast his line and we sat. We sat for what seemed like hours, but I knew only a few short minutes had passed. The sun was beating down on us. Maybe it was the time of day, maybe the circumstances at the time, but it was a much different sun than I had encountered that morning. The heat was unbearable. I began to feel extremely uncomfortable.

I exchanged nervous glances with Eileen.

"He's in pain," Eileen mouthed to me.

"Should we take him back?" I mouthed in response.

We decided to stay put for a while and give it some more time. The club members continued to visit with us, one at a time, in between casts. At one point, Bill motioned for Christian to take hold of his line.

"I think this one is a lucky one, Christian. I just have a feeling about it."

No sooner did Christian take hold than the line gave a jerk.

"Hey! Would you look at that? You've got a fish on that line! Reel it in! Reel it in, Christian!"

Christian reeled in the fish, but there was no fooling him. Though an old soul in a young boy's body, he was tickled by their gesture. He reeled the fish in, never letting on that he knew what they had done. The men were beaming. They took a picture of Christian with *his* fish. They gave him a certificate, indicating exactly what type of fish he caught. Then they gave him a dollar for the catch.

"Christian, we make it a policy to give a dollar for each fish caught on the pier. I have a feeling you're going to take us to the bank today!"

As our morning on the pier progressed the men continued to hand off their lines to Christian. Each took turns offering soda, ice cream, and chips. One gentleman even took time away from his lines to come over and show Christian some paper tricks. An old newspaper was made into a Christmas tree. A white flyer became a boat. Seeing a definite connection between this man's paper folding and our cranes, Eileen and I immediately lit up. Christian, however, remained hunched over, in fetal position, without so much as a trace of a smile on his face.

Before long, it was after noon and I decided to venture back to the house to get some lunch for Eileen and Christian. My mind was racing. All I wanted was for Christian to have a good time. It didn't appear that he was. The boy who always smiled wasn't smiling. He looked miserable. I said a quick prayer.

Upon my return, I couldn't believe my eyes! Not only was Christian smiling, asking questions, and talking, he was up out of his wheelchair! In nothing but his socks, Christian was practically running from side to side on that pier, pointing down into the water!

"Look, Mom-Mom! I found some! I found a whole school of fish!"

And so he did. He found school after school of fish. The pictures were taken. The certificates were filled out and Christian was given dollar after dollar after dollar. Even though the fish were not large ones, they were Christian's fish. He had caught them entirely on his own.

The club members started a bucket for Christian. Each fish he caught was placed into that bucket. A younger gentleman asked if he could use one of Christian's fish as live bait. Christian was thrilled. You should have seen the look on his face. He really was a member of the Fishing Club.

By the time we left the pier that day, Christian was calling every member by name. What's more, he had used every single one of their poles. After all, that's what members do! We left with an open invitation to come back and fish with them any time of day, any day of the week. I could not thank them enough.

On my way out, I placed a small paper crane on the desk of the clubhouse. Although they had not been there to fold with us, they had definitely become honorary members of our Cranes for Christian Community.

ANOTHER PHONE CALL

No one who visited Christian in the coming weeks was permitted to leave without seeing his Ocean Grove pictures. He was so proud, so happy with his experience. Yes, that fishing trip got Christian through some very dark days. Whenever he was feeling down, all he needed to do was take out his little photo album. Eileen says it was one of his fondest memories.

As summer ended and the new school year approached, we all started to make our preparations. I went in to set up my third grade classroom. Eileen took Christian for a visit to the middle school. We were still unsure as to whether or not Christian would be well enough to attend. Turns out, he was not well enough. He never went.

Christian's cousin Kajai was with us at School Five though. A third grader now, Eileen talked to me about the possibility of placing her in my room. As much as I loved Kajai, I didn't think it was a good idea. I suggested another placement. No one wanted to discuss it, but we all knew the time was coming. Christian would not be with us much longer. I wanted Kajai's time at school to be an escape; I wanted school to be the one place that took her away from it all.

Seeing me would only be a constant reminder. Eileen was hesitant at first, but she later agreed.

I assured Eileen, "If she ever needs me, I'm right across the hallway. She can come and spend time with me in my classroom."

Together with the building principal and Kajai's third grade teacher, an open door policy was adopted. Most of the time Kajai and I just waved to each other in passing and that was enough. Other times, a hug was needed to make it through the day.

Our open door policy was not put into full effect until late September. While leaving the media center after a third grade presentation, Kajai approached me. One minute it was a smile and a hug, the next minute it was sobbing and a tear-stained face!

"Did you hear about our Christian? He's going to die, Mrs. Sirdashney. He's going to die!"

I motioned to my grade level partners. It was time for third grade specials. One of them took my class to the gym. Kajai stayed with me as her class went to music.

It was true. Christian was going to die. He was placed on hospice, his care and level of pain now being too extensive for Eileen to manage on her own. How much time did he have left? No one knew for sure. Each and every additional day was a gift for us, but a tremendous struggle for Christian.

Kajai and I made our way back to my classroom. I invited

her inside. As we sat at the reading table together that day, I realized for the first time how very much Kajai resembled her cousin. Yes, she had his kind and quiet nature, but my goodness! Sitting across the reading table from her, it was as if I was indeed with Christian. Her eyes ... Her voice ... Her cheeks ... They were just like Christian's. She was Christian in his healthier days. She was Christian when he was with me years prior, and she was sitting in his special seat.

Kajai visited my classroom several times that school year. Sometimes she just needed to take a walk over to say a quick hello. Other times she stayed for quite a while. It was a difficult time for all of us, let alone the children and especially Kajai. Christian and Kajai shared a very special bond. He was her protector. I knew he would want me to watch over her at School Five. I would continue to do so as long as I was needed. Little did I know what watching over Kajai would entail in a very few short days to come.

It was an afternoon in mid-October, and I was called to the School Five office. Another teacher was sent to watch my class, so up I went. I know it sounds silly, especially being an elementary school teacher now, but I still associate the office with being in trouble. I was actually nervous walking the hallways!

Mary and Cheryl, two office assistants and good friends of mine, awaited my arrival. The principal was standing in the door of her private office, motioning for me to come in. The look on their faces, especially Mary and Cheryl, whom I had known for so long, was chilling! My heart plummeted.

"What? What happened? Is it Mike? Is it Faith?"

My body was trembling. I could barely breathe.

Mary and Cheryl opened their mouths to speak, but nothing came out. Tears filled their eyes. Mrs. Lupia put her arm around me and brought me into her office. The door closed. Waiting inside for me was the school counselor and the school nurse.

"Erica, Eileen just called. Christian's gone."

Oh, my dear Lord ... I was shocked. I know we were told any time now, but the thought of losing him that day never even crossed my mind!

"But I was just with him last night! I saw him! He was fine! He was eating!"

And I *had* just seen him the night before. Christian called and asked if I could come over. Mike, Faith, and I picked up some food, movies, and treats and we spent the majority of the day with him and his family.

"He had a cheeseburger and two packages of apple dippers! He asked for more! He had seconds! How could he be gone?"

I'm sure to the others I sounded like a raving lunatic. Why was I going on and on about food? What difference did it make? Well, it made a *big* difference. The doctors told us when it was Christian's time there would be signs for us to watch for. One of the major signs was he would no longer eat or drink. I think I really took this to heart. It became my primary focus. If Christian was eating, I felt confident when I said good-bye. He was going to be okay. I'd see him another day.

I said good-bye to him that night, just as I had done countless other times. He was lying on the floor in considerable amount of pain, but I was confident he would be okay. He had walked with me, talked with me, watched movies, and laughed with me all day long. Most importantly, he ate! I could say good-bye to him that night because he ate. That was the rule, the rule I had set within the confines of my heart and mind.

How could he be gone? As I began to think about it more, however, things started to fall into place. Talking to Eileen about it later that day helped as well. Yes, Christian ate. He ate because Mrs. Sirdashney was there. He ate because that was what he always did for Mrs. Sirdashney. Sometimes he ate because it made him feel better; most times he ate because it made *her* feel better. That amazing little soul!

Hadn't he planned his last day so perfectly? Didn't he make it a point to reach out to and visit with each and every person who was special to him? This was his way of saying good-bye. He was saying thank you. He was saying I love you to each and every one of us. It was exactly what

Christian wanted. He even had a sleepover with his cousins! A sleepover they were begging for, for ages, but Christian never felt up to it. Well, they had their sleepover. Christian, Jamal and Kajai.

"Oh my goodness, Kajai! Where is Kajai? Has anyone told her?"

Kajai was still in class. No one had told her. No one was coming for her. I called Eileen.

"Would you tell her, Erica? Would you tell her and bring her home? He's still here. Come say good-bye."

I was given a few minutes to get myself together and gather my thoughts. Then Kajai was sent for and they led her into the office where I was now the one waiting. The one with the news.

Kajai was petrified. An honor roll student, and one who is always well behaved, she too associated the office with being in trouble. We all greeted her with extra big smiles. Upon entering the principal's office, the door closed once again. I motioned for Kajai to come over by me. She grabbed my hand as I invited her to sit on my lap. Her head tucked into my shoulder instinctively.

"We had a great time together with Christian yesterday, didn't we?"

"Yeah, we did."

"And you finally got to have your sleepover with the boys. Wasn't that terrific?"

"I know. I didn't know if we ever would."

"Well, you did and I'm so glad you did. Christian's glad you did too, because he loves you so much and he wants you to be happy."

"Christian wants everyone to be happy, Mrs. Sirdashney."

"Yes, I know, sweetie. That's one of the reasons why Christian is so special. He wants everyone to be happy and he does whatever it takes to make people happy. Even when he's not... Even when he's sick... Even when he's in so, so much pain. Sweetie, Christian's not in pain anymore. He's is heaven with God. Christian died today."

Her only response was, "Oh my..."

She sat on my lap for a considerable amount of time. I hugged her and I told her I was sorry. I kept repeating the fact that Christian was not in pain anymore. He loved us and we loved him. Because of our love for him, we didn't want him to be in pain anymore. As much as we missed him and wished he didn't have to go, we would be happy for him because he was no longer in pain. She nodded as I spoke, agreeing with all that I said.

I asked Kajai if she was ready to go home. Her family was waiting for her. Christian was waiting for her, and we were going to go say good-bye. Kajai's things were gathered from her classroom and we left School Five to go say good-bye to Christian.

SAYING GOOD-BYE

Many family members were waiting for Kajai when we arrived. She went ahead with them. I lagged behind. Most of the faces I did not recognize. I did not know who these people were. Perhaps they did not know me either. I began to question my being there. Eileen said to come, but was it really my place? I didn't want to upset anyone. I didn't want to intrude.

People gathered outside the front door. The stairway was packed, as was the living room, dining room, kitchen, and patio. I made my way through the crowd of young and old. I found my way to Eileen. She embraced me.

"Thank you so much!" she said. "Thank you!"

I sat with Eileen on the couch for a while. I asked how she was doing. She told me about Christian. She told me about his passing. She was handling it all considerably well.

"How can I be upset, Erica? He's not in pain anymore! He's up there saying no more pain, Mom-Mom! Look at me! No more medicine, Mom-Mom!"

We talked about his last day with all of us.

"He knew, Erica. He knew exactly what he needed to do

and he knew exactly whom he needed to see before he could go. Speaking of which ..."

Eileen told me it was time to say good-bye.

"He's still here. He's at peace. It's a peaceful sleep he so rarely had these days. You know what that looks like though, don't you. It's okay. Go and say good-bye."

I made my way through the crowd in the hallway and waited as people gathered around his bedside. Groups of people continued to gather in the bedroom, but the bedside was no longer occupied. I approached the bed and knelt down beside him.

"Hi, buddy."

I silently prayed at Christian's bedside. Then I kissed him on the forehead and said good-bye.

I made my way back to Eileen and sat with her for a bit longer. However, it wasn't long until her attention shifted elsewhere. Her one son was due to arrive any time now. She was fearful of his reaction, fearful of how he would take the news. Her pastor consoled her and stood guard awaiting the son's arrival.

I sat on the couch by myself, taking it all in. Kajai joined me for a brief time. She had made it her goal to care for Christian's small dog now that he was gone. I helped her find some dog food in the kitchen. That's where I ran into a former student from School Five. Ebony, a beautiful girl inside and out, was at School Five with me years ago. She was not in my class, but she remembered me and I remembered her. We talked for a while.

Before long, a terrible feeling overpowered me. I was having difficulty breathing. My emotional state had triggered an asthma attack. I went out on the balcony to get some air. The few people present eyed me cautiously as I coughed. One by one they went back inside until I was left with one individual remaining. I reached in my bag for my inhaler.

"Are you okay?" she asked

"I think so, thank you."

Awkward silence.

"Are you Lisa?"

I thought I overheard someone call her by name. I never met her, but I knew of her. She was like a godmother to Christian.

"Yes, I'm Lisa."

"Hi, Lisa, I'm Erica Sirdashney. I was…"

But before I could continue explaining who I was, Lisa said, "I know exactly who you are."

Her tone of voice made it difficult to determine whether or not that was a good thing or a bad thing. Was I correct in thinking I had no place being there? Was I intruding? Were people looking at me, thinking, *Who is she? What is she doing here?*

Perhaps Lisa could sense my vulnerability. Perhaps she knew what I was thinking that very moment because she reached over and hugged me. Into my ear she whispered, "You know I used to be his favorite."

So, I was wrong. Boy, was I wrong! All of my insecurities, all of my fears. I was not intruding. This is where I was meant to be. And how amazing that such a diverse group of people could come together. Different races, different ages, different walks of life. None of it mattered. We were all there. We were all together. And what brought us together? The love of a little boy. Our love for a little boy. An old soul in a young boy's body!

The world could learn a lot from our Christian.

CRANES FROM CHRISTIAN

I made my way home. As I pulled into my development I remember catching a glimpse of the evening sky. The sun was just about setting, nestled behind a cluster of beautiful fluffy white clouds. The rays of light shot out in every direction. I cannot remember a time the sky looked more beautiful! It was a heavenly sight. I just knew Christian was shining down upon us all.

My husband was waiting for me in the driveway. Once again contacted by my family at Five, he greeted me with a smile and a hug.

"I'm so sorry," were his only words.

Dinner was cheerful, as my four-year-old daughter was busy telling us about her day. I knew I'd have to tell her about Christian. I dreaded doing so. Mike and I decided to wait until after dinner.

Christian and Faith too shared a special bond. She adored him and he adored her. After all, they had a lot in common. Both the strong, silent type; they don't say much, but what they say, they mean. And they're loyal to the ones they love.

Never was this more apparent than after one of our family visits to CHOP. No sooner were we out the door, than

Christian turned to Eileen and said, "You know, Mom-Mom? I really like that Faith."

Unfortunately, Eileen did not fully hear what he had said. She kept questioning,

"What? Who? I don't know what you're talking about Christian."

"Faith, Mom-Mom. Faith! You don't know who Faith is, Mom-Mom? She was just here with Mr. and Mrs. Sirdashney! There's something seriously wrong with you, Mom-Mom. I think you need to go to the doctor!"

To this day, that's one of our favorite stories. We tell it over and over again. I love it because it shows how much Christian cared for Faith. I love it because it shows how much Christian worried about Eileen. I love it because it shows what a tremendous spirit Christian had and what a terrific kid he was. Most of all, I love it because Eileen laughs hysterically every time she retells it. Oh! The gifts he has left us.

So yes, it was time to tell Faith about Christian. We washed up for bed, put pajamas on, read a story, and said our prayers. After prayers I told Faith Christian was in heaven. I told her Christian died and he was one of God's angels now.

Her response was quite strange. Not really paying attention to what I was saying, Faith looked past me and started to giggle. Mike tried to intervene, repeating much of what

I said, but she looked straight past him too, giggling louder and louder!

"He's so funny, Mommy."

"Who's funny, sweetie?"

"Christian is Mommy. He's just so funny!"

"What do you mean Christian's funny?"

"He says blub-blub-blah-blah-blah-blah-blub! Blub-blub
-blah-blah-blah-blah-blub!"

Faith continued making faces at the ceiling, giggling and chanting the same silly nonsense phrase over and over again. Mike and I looked back over the past couple of days, searching for a logical explanation of what was taking place. However, this was not something Christian had done neither at the hospital, nor during one of our visits at each other's homes. Where was she getting this? According to Faith, Christian was there and he was doing it that very moment!

When I relayed the story to Eileen the following day, she burst out in laughter.

"I don't doubt it, Erica. I don't doubt it. That's exactly what he would do. He may not have been in any condition to do so in the time he knew her on earth, but I don't doubt that he's up there doing it now!"

What an amazing child! I cannot say that enough!

He was an amazing child. Christian was so amazing that he planned his entire funeral service. Shortly before his passing, he sat with his pastor and talked about what he wanted. Not for himself, but for others.

"I don't want people to be sad. I want them to be happy. I want people to sing. I want people to dance. I want them to rejoice," he said.

Flowers were something else Christian didn't want.

"No flowers!"

So we didn't do flowers. We did *cranes*!

At Eileen's request I picked up the cranes, all 1,000, and I brought them back to my house. One by one I clipped their strings and removed them from the beautiful strands. One by one I pinned them on wreaths, placed them in treasure boxes, and decorated a banner that read, "Christian, Forever in our Hearts!"

Arrangements were made with the church. Mike and I went over the night before the service to set up. It drew quite a crowd. Help was offered. Questions were asked. People started making new cranes. Tables were set up with Christian's cranes, his prized possessions, and pictures of his loved ones. It was beautiful. Anyone could see how much this child was loved. Anyone could see how he brought a whole community of people together.

At the entrance of the church there was a portrait of Christian. He was terribly ill and in considerable amount of pain at the time the photo was taken. But that didn't stop him smiling from ear to ear. He was simply beaming! Next to the photo was a large basket of cranes with a new poem. You see; Cranes for Christian had become Cranes from Christian. The poem read:

CRANES FROM CHRISTIAN

An angel in the heavens,
He shines from up above.
Please take a crane and keep it
as a symbol of his *love*!

We sang that day. We danced. We rejoiced. The service was absolutely beautiful. People spoke. People read poetry. A slideshow was displayed on a large screen. There were pictures of Christian as an infant, pictures of him as a toddler, pictures with Mom-Mom, pictures with his cousins, then there was a picture that caused me to cry out in such a way, I almost didn't even recognize the sound of my own voice!

It was the picture of Christian in Ocean Grove. A picture of Christian sleeping so soundly... The makings of that trademark smile about to emerge. This was *my* picture, *my* memory. I remembered taking it. I remembered the experience we shared and I was overcome. I sobbed uncontrollably.

I sobbed not out of grief, but out of joy. Christian was no longer in pain. He was home. He was happy and I was happy for him. I was grateful for the time we had together, the influence he had on my life. I was indeed loved, and his love made me a better person. The world could indeed learn a lot from our little Christian. The world could learn a lot!

The service ended with an answering machine message Christian had left for his pastor a few days prior. He said, "Hi … It's Christian … I love you … Good-bye …"

Perhaps this was another case of Christian knowing exactly what he was doing and why. Yes, this was indeed Christian's good-bye to us all.

E rica, do you think we would have been able to do any of this for Christian if we had another child now?"

That was the question my husband asked as we were leaving CHOP one day after a visit with Christian, and the answer was *no*. If we had another child when we wanted to, when we planned to do so, we probably would not have been in a position to reach out to Christian and his family the way that we did. We wouldn't have had the time. We wouldn't have had the resources. In fact who's to say I would have even been at School Five to teach the year Christian was in third grade?

Our battle with infertility was a long one, a painful one. The situation was such that a doctor once told us *Faith* was a beautiful name, but we should have named our daughter *Miracle*. Doctors had no idea how we were able to conceive, but one thing was certain. It was highly unlikely we'd ever be able to conceive again. The thought of that broke our hearts. But then again, what's that phrase? *Everything happens for a reason!*

Yes, once again, everything happens for a reason. There

may have been a number of reasons for our inability to conceive. However, if Christian was the one and only, I was more than happy to accept it. This was clearly part of God's plan. I took comfort in knowing. Knowing was indeed a privilege.

Shortly after Christian's death Eileen said to me, "You will have another child, Erica. You will. Mark my words. You will have another child and it will be a *boy*! Christian's going to help hand pick that little soul who comes to bless your lives. You wait. You'll see!"

Nicholas Christian was born on February 7, 2007. And do you know what? He's got a great smile!

Thanks, Christian. I miss you, buddy!